FAST FEAST REPEAT

Cookbook

Step-by-Step Guide to Reset Your Metabolism, Lose Weight and Embracing a Balanced Lifestyle with Intermittent Fasting.

Mariyam Mohl

TABLE OF CONTENT

INTRODUCTION

Join us on a gastronomic adventure that honors a simple, health-conscious living through the "Fast Feast Repeat Cookbook." This cookbook is based on the ideas of Delay, Don't Deny Intermittent Fasting, which combines the joy of enjoying healthful, delicious meals with the skill of balance.

You will find a selection of recipes in these pages that have been thoughtfully created to go along with your intermittent fasting adventure. Regardless of your experience level with time-restricted eating, this cookbook is meant to make your feasting periods fulfilling, your fasting days delectable, and the repetition of this well-balanced lifestyle both doable and pleasurable.

We are aware that adopting an intermittent fasting lifestyle involves developing a sustainable and pleasurable relationship with food in addition to providing your body with nourishment. "Fast Feast Repeat Cookbook" gives you the tools to make mindful decisions and offers a variety of delicious recipes that make every meal a joyful occasion, whether you're feasting or fasting.

Every meal, from filling dinners to vigorous breakfasts, has been carefully chosen to provide your body with the nutrition it requires, improve your experience fasting, and promote your general health. The cookbook is your reliable companion on the road to a healthier and more mindful lifestyle since it combines scientifically supported advice with creative cooking.

Come embrace the Fast. Feast. Repeat. pattern, in which each mouthful serves as a chance to nourish, indulge, and recognize the progress made toward a better, more fulfilling version of yourself. Take off on a delectable journey of self-discovery and culinary exploration with the "Fast Feast Repeat Cookbook" as your guide. One healthy meal at a time, here's to enjoying life to the fullest!

Green Smoothie Bowl

Ingredients:

- 1 cup spinach (fresh or frozen)
- 1/2 banana (frozen for a thicker consistency)
- 1/2 avocado
- 1/2 cup unsweetened almond milk (or any preferred milk)
- 1 tablespoon chia seeds
- 1 tablespoon almond butter
- Toppings: Sliced kiwi, berries, granola, pumpkin seeds, shredded coconut

Instructions:

1. In a blender, combine spinach, banana, avocado, almond milk, chia seeds, and almond butter.
2. Blend until smooth and creamy, adding more almond milk if needed to reach your desired consistency.
3. Pour the green smoothie into a bowl.

Toppings: 4. Arrange sliced kiwi, berries, granola, pumpkin seeds, and shredded coconut on top.

Benefits:

- **Nutrient-Dense:** Packed with vitamins and minerals from spinach, banana, and berries.
- **Healthy Fats:** Avocado and almond butter provide monounsaturated fats for sustained energy.

- **Hydration:** Almond milk contributes to hydration without added sugars found in some other beverages.
- **Fiber Boost:** Chia seeds and the variety of toppings add fiber, promoting digestive health.
- **Antioxidants:** Berries and spinach are rich in antioxidants that support overall well-being.

Application:

1. **Breakfast Boost:** Enjoy the green smoothie bowl as a nutritious and energizing breakfast.
2. **Post-Workout Recovery:** The combination of protein-rich almond butter and chia seeds makes this bowl a great post-workout option.
3. **Snack Attack:** Satisfy afternoon cravings with a refreshing and filling green smoothie bowl.
4. **Customizable Treat:** Experiment with different toppings and variations based on personal taste preferences and dietary needs.

Cauliflower Crust Margherita Pizza

Ingredients: *For the Cauliflower Crust:*

- 1 medium-sized cauliflower head, riced (about 3 cups)
- 1 egg
- 1 cup shredded mozzarella cheese
- 1 teaspoon dried oregano
- 1/2 teaspoon garlic powder
- Salt and pepper to taste

For the Margherita Toppings:

- 1/2 cup tomato sauce
- 1-2 medium-sized tomatoes, sliced
- 1 cup fresh mozzarella, sliced
- Fresh basil leaves
- Olive oil for drizzling

Instructions:

Cauliflower Crust:

1. Preheat your oven to 400°F (200°C).
2. Rice the cauliflower by using a food processor or grater.
3. Microwave the riced cauliflower for 4-5 minutes or until softened. Allow it to cool.
4. Place the cooled cauliflower in a clean kitchen towel and wring out excess moisture.
5. In a bowl, combine the cauliflower, egg, shredded mozzarella, oregano, garlic powder, salt, and pepper. Mix until a dough forms.

6. Spread the cauliflower dough onto a parchment-lined baking sheet, forming a pizza crust shape.
7. Bake the crust for 20-25 minutes or until golden brown and firm.

Assembling the Margherita Pizza: 8. Once the crust is ready, spread tomato sauce evenly over the surface.

9. Add sliced tomatoes and fresh mozzarella on top.
10. Bake for an additional 10-15 minutes or until the cheese is melted and bubbly.
11. Remove from the oven and garnish with fresh basil leaves.
12. Drizzle with olive oil just before serving.

Benefits:

- **Low Carb Alternative:** Cauliflower crust is a low-carb and gluten-free option, suitable for those with dietary restrictions.
- **Rich in Vegetables:** The pizza is loaded with fresh tomatoes and basil, providing essential vitamins and antioxidants.
- **Moderate Healthy Fats:** Mozzarella and olive oil offer a satisfying dose of healthy fats.
- **Calorie Control:** Compared to traditional pizza crusts, cauliflower crust is often lower in calories.

Application:
1. **Family Dinner Night:** Make pizza night healthier by serving Cauliflower Crust Margherita Pizza.
2. **Entertaining Guests:** Impress friends and family with a homemade, gourmet-style pizza.
3. **Lunch or Dinner Option:** Enjoy this pizza as a satisfying lunch or dinner that's both delicious and nutritious.
4. **Customization:** Experiment with additional toppings like olives, spinach, or grilled chicken for variety.

Lemon Garlic Shrimp Zoodles

Ingredients:

- 1 pound large shrimp, peeled and deveined
- 4 medium zucchinis, spiralized into zoodles
- 3 tablespoons olive oil
- 4 cloves garlic, minced
- Zest of 1 lemon
- Juice of 1 lemon
- 1 teaspoon red pepper flakes (optional for heat)
- Salt and pepper to taste
- Fresh parsley, chopped (for garnish)

Instructions:

1. **Prepare Shrimp:**
   - In a large skillet, heat 2 tablespoons of olive oil over medium-high heat.
   - Add shrimp and cook until they turn pink, about 2-3 minutes per side. Remove the shrimp from the skillet and set aside.

2. **Cook Zoodles:**
   - In the same skillet, add the remaining tablespoon of olive oil.
   - Add minced garlic and sauté for 1-2 minutes until fragrant but not browned.
   - Add the spiralized zucchini (zoodles) to the skillet and sauté for

2-3 minutes until just tender but not mushy.

3. **Combine:**
   - Return the cooked shrimp to the skillet with the zoodles.
   - Add lemon zest, lemon juice, red pepper flakes (if using), salt, and pepper. Toss everything together until well combined and heated through.

4. **Serve:**
   - Divide the lemon garlic shrimp and zoodles among plates.
   - Garnish with fresh chopped parsley.

Benefits:
- **Low-Calorie Option:** Zoodles are a low-calorie alternative to traditional pasta, making this dish lighter.
- **High Protein:** Shrimp is a lean source of protein, promoting muscle health.
- **Rich in Vitamin C:** Lemon adds a burst of vitamin C, supporting the immune system.
- **Healthy Fats:** Olive oil provides monounsaturated fats that are beneficial for heart health.

Application:
1. **Quick Weeknight Dinner:** Lemon Garlic Shrimp Zoodles make for a quick and healthy weeknight meal that's ready in under 30 minutes.

2. **Light Lunch:** Enjoy as a satisfying and light lunch option.
3. **Meal Prep:** Prepare a batch for meal prepping and enjoy throughout the week.
4. **Guest-Worthy Dish:** Impress guests with this flavorful and visually appealing dish at dinner parties.

Cabbage and Sausage Skillet

Ingredients:

- 1 pound smoked sausage, sliced
- 1 medium cabbage, shredded
- 1 onion, thinly sliced
- 2 cloves garlic, minced
- 2 tablespoons olive oil
- 1 teaspoon paprika
- Salt and pepper to taste
- Fresh parsley, chopped (for garnish)

Instructions:

1. **Sauté Sausage:**
   - In a large skillet, heat olive oil over medium-high heat.
   - Add sliced sausage and cook until browned on both sides. Remove the sausage from the skillet and set aside.

2. **Sauté Vegetables:**
   - In the same skillet, add sliced onion and minced garlic. Sauté until softened and aromatic.
   - Add shredded cabbage to the skillet and cook for 5-7 minutes, or until the cabbage is tender-crisp.

3. **Combine:**
   - Return the cooked sausage to the skillet with the cabbage and onions.

- Sprinkle paprika over the mixture and toss everything together until well combined.

4. **Season and Garnish:**
   - Season with salt and pepper to taste.
   - Garnish with chopped fresh parsley.

Benefits:
- **High in Fiber:** Cabbage is rich in fiber, aiding in digestion and promoting gut health.
- **Protein Source:** Smoked sausage provides a flavorful protein source.
- **Nutrient-Rich:** Cabbage contains vitamins C and K, and antioxidants that contribute to overall well-being.
- **Quick and Easy:** This one-pan dish is quick to prepare, making it perfect for busy weeknights.

Application:
1. **Weeknight Dinner:** Cabbage and Sausage Skillet is a quick and satisfying dinner option for busy evenings.
2. **Meal Prep:** Make a larger batch for meal prepping and divide into containers for easy lunches throughout the week.
3. **Comfort Food:** Enjoy the warm and hearty flavors of this skillet dish during colder seasons.

4. **Potluck or Gathering:** Serve at potlucks or family gatherings as a crowd-pleasing, flavorful side dish.

Spinach and Feta Stuffed Chicken Breast

Ingredients:
- 4 boneless, skinless chicken breasts
- 2 cups fresh spinach, chopped
- 1 cup feta cheese, crumbled
- 1 tablespoon olive oil
- 2 cloves garlic, minced
- 1 teaspoon dried oregano
- Salt and pepper to taste
- Toothpicks or kitchen twine (for securing)

Instructions:
1. **Preheat Oven:**
   - Preheat the oven to 375°F (190°C).
2. **Prepare Chicken:**
   - Lay each chicken breast flat on a cutting board.
   - Carefully slice a pocket into each chicken breast, ensuring not to cut through the other side.
3. **Make Filling:**
   - In a skillet, heat olive oil over medium heat.
   - Add minced garlic and sauté until fragrant.
   - Add chopped spinach and cook until wilted.
   - Remove from heat and stir in crumbled feta cheese, oregano, salt, and pepper.

4. **Stuff Chicken:**
   - Stuff each chicken breast pocket with the spinach and feta mixture, securing the openings with toothpicks or by tying with kitchen twine.
5. **Sear Chicken:**
   - In an oven-safe skillet, heat a bit of olive oil over medium-high heat.
   - Sear the stuffed chicken breasts on each side until golden brown.
6. **Bake:**
   - Transfer the skillet to the preheated oven and bake for 20-25 minutes or until the chicken reaches an internal temperature of 165°F (74°C).
7. **Serve:**
   - Remove toothpicks or twine before serving.
   - Optionally, drizzle with pan juices and garnish with fresh herbs.

Benefits:
- **High Protein:** Chicken breast provides a lean source of protein, essential for muscle health.
- **Iron and Calcium:** Spinach offers iron, while feta contributes calcium for bone health.
- **Healthy Fats:** Olive oil and feta provide monounsaturated fats that support heart health.

- **Vitamins and Minerals:** Spinach is rich in vitamins A, C, and K, and various minerals.

Application:

1. **Dinner Entree:** Serve Spinach and Feta Stuffed Chicken Breast as a delicious and elegant main course for dinner.
2. **Date Night:** Impress your partner with a restaurant-quality dish for a special date night at home.
3. **Family Gathering:** Make a larger batch for a family gathering or holiday meal.
4. **Meal Prep:** Prepare in advance for a week of tasty and nutritious lunches.

Eggplant and Zucchini Lasagna

Ingredients:

- 1 large eggplant, thinly sliced lengthwise
- 2 medium zucchinis, thinly sliced lengthwise
- 1 pound ground turkey or beef (optional)
- 1 onion, finely chopped
- 3 cloves garlic, minced
- 1 can (28 oz) crushed tomatoes
- 2 cups ricotta cheese
- 1 cup shredded mozzarella cheese
- 1/2 cup grated Parmesan cheese
- 1 egg
- 2 tablespoons olive oil
- 1 teaspoon dried oregano
- 1 teaspoon dried basil
- Salt and pepper to taste
- Fresh basil or parsley for garnish

Instructions:

1. **Preheat Oven:**
   - Preheat the oven to 375°F (190°C).
2. **Prepare Vegetables:**
   - Lay out the sliced eggplant and zucchini on paper towels. Sprinkle with salt and let sit for 15-20 minutes to release excess moisture. Pat dry with paper towels.

3. **Brown Meat (Optional):**
   - In a skillet, heat olive oil over medium heat.
   - Add chopped onion and garlic, sauté until softened.
   - If using ground meat, add it to the skillet and cook until browned. Drain excess fat.
4. **Prepare Tomato Sauce:**
   - Add crushed tomatoes, oregano, basil, salt, and pepper to the skillet. Simmer for 10-15 minutes.
5. **Prepare Cheese Mixture:**
   - In a bowl, mix ricotta cheese, mozzarella, Parmesan, and egg until well combined.
6. **Assemble Lasagna:**
   - In a greased baking dish, spread a layer of tomato sauce.
   - Layer with slices of eggplant and zucchini.
   - Add a layer of the meat mixture (if using) and then a layer of the cheese mixture.
   - Repeat the layers until ingredients are used, finishing with a layer of cheese on top.
7. **Bake:**
   - Cover the baking dish with foil and bake for 30 minutes.

- Remove the foil and bake for an additional 15-20 minutes until the top is golden and bubbly.

8. **Serve:**
   - Allow the lasagna to cool for a few minutes before slicing.
   - Garnish with fresh basil or parsley before serving.

Benefits:
- **Vegetable-Rich:** Eggplant and zucchini add vitamins, minerals, and fiber to the dish.
- **Protein Source:** Ground turkey or beef provides a protein boost.
- **Calcium and Protein:** Ricotta and mozzarella contribute calcium and protein for bone health and muscle support.
- **Antioxidants:** Tomato sauce is rich in antioxidants, promoting overall health.

Application:
1. **Family Dinner:** Eggplant and Zucchini Lasagna makes for a wholesome family dinner.
2. **Vegetarian Option:** Omit the meat for a delicious vegetarian lasagna.
3. **Meal Prep:** Prepare in advance and enjoy leftovers throughout the week.
4. **Potluck or Gathering:** Bring this hearty dish to potlucks or family gatherings.

Roasted Brussels Sprouts with Balsamic Glaze

Ingredients:

- 1 pound Brussels sprouts, trimmed and halved
- 2 tablespoons olive oil
- Salt and pepper to taste
- 2 tablespoons balsamic vinegar
- 1 tablespoon honey or maple syrup (optional, for sweetness)
- 1-2 cloves garlic, minced (optional, for added flavor)
- 2 tablespoons grated Parmesan cheese (optional, for garnish)
- Chopped fresh parsley or thyme for garnish

Instructions:

1. **Preheat Oven:**
   - Preheat the oven to 400°F (200°C).
2. **Prepare Brussels Sprouts:**
   - Trim the ends of Brussels sprouts and cut them in half.
3. **Season and Toss:**
   - In a bowl, toss Brussels sprouts with olive oil, salt, and pepper until evenly coated.
4. **Roast Brussels Sprouts:**
   - Spread the Brussels sprouts in a single layer on a baking sheet.

- Roast in the preheated oven for 20-25 minutes or until they are golden brown and crispy on the edges, tossing halfway through for even cooking.

5. **Prepare Balsamic Glaze:**
   - While the Brussels sprouts are roasting, in a small saucepan, heat balsamic vinegar over medium heat.
   - If desired, add honey or maple syrup for sweetness and minced garlic for extra flavor.
   - Simmer for 5-7 minutes or until the glaze thickens slightly.

6. **Toss in Glaze:**
   - Once the Brussels sprouts are done roasting, transfer them to a bowl.
   - Drizzle the balsamic glaze over the roasted Brussels sprouts and toss to coat evenly.

7. **Serve:**
   - Transfer to a serving dish, garnish with grated Parmesan cheese (if using), and sprinkle with fresh parsley or thyme.

Benefits:
- **High in Fiber:** Brussels sprouts are rich in fiber, promoting digestive health.

- **Vitamins and Minerals:** Brussels sprouts contain vitamins C and K, and various minerals.
- **Antioxidant-Rich:** Balsamic vinegar provides antioxidants that contribute to overall well-being.
- **Heart-Healthy Fats:** Olive oil contributes monounsaturated fats, supporting heart health.

Application:

1. **Side Dish:** Serve Roasted Brussels Sprouts with Balsamic Glaze as a flavorful side dish for any meal.
2. **Appetizer:** Present them as a delicious appetizer for gatherings or dinner parties.
3. **Salad Topping:** Add these roasted Brussels sprouts to salads for a unique and tasty twist.
4. **Meal Prep:** Prepare a batch for meal prepping and enjoy throughout the week.

Vegetarian Chili with Black Beans

Ingredients:

- 2 cans (15 oz each) black beans, drained and rinsed
- 1 can (28 oz) diced tomatoes, undrained
- 1 cup corn kernels (fresh, frozen, or canned)
- 1 large bell pepper, diced
- 1 large onion, diced
- 3 cloves garlic, minced
- 2 tablespoons olive oil
- 1 jalapeño, diced (optional, for heat)
- 2 tablespoons chili powder
- 1 teaspoon ground cumin
- 1 teaspoon smoked paprika
- 1/2 teaspoon cayenne pepper (adjust to taste, for extra heat)
- Salt and pepper to taste
- 2 cups vegetable broth
- 1 cup tomato sauce
- Juice of 1 lime
- Fresh cilantro for garnish
- Avocado slices for topping (optional)

Instructions:

1. **Sauté Vegetables:**
   - In a large pot, heat olive oil over medium heat.

- Add diced onion, bell pepper, and garlic. Sauté until vegetables are softened.

2. **Spice it Up:**
   - Stir in chili powder, cumin, smoked paprika, and cayenne pepper (if using). Cook for an additional 1-2 minutes to toast the spices.

3. **Add Beans and Tomatoes:**
   - Add black beans, diced tomatoes, and corn to the pot.
   - Pour in vegetable broth and tomato sauce. Stir well to combine.

4. **Simmer:**
   - Bring the chili to a simmer, then reduce the heat to low. Cover and let it simmer for 20-25 minutes, allowing flavors to meld.

5. **Adjust Seasoning:**
   - Season with salt and pepper to taste. Adjust the chili powder or cayenne pepper for more heat if desired.

6. **Finish and Serve:**
   - Stir in lime juice just before serving.
   - Ladle the chili into bowls and garnish with fresh cilantro. Top with avocado slices if desired.

Benefits:
- **Plant-Based Protein:** Black beans provide a hearty source of plant-based protein.
- **Fiber-Rich:** Beans and vegetables contribute to the chili's high fiber content, supporting digestive health.
- **Vitamins and Antioxidants:** Bell peppers, tomatoes, and onions offer essential vitamins and antioxidants.
- **Low in Saturated Fat:** Being vegetarian, this chili is naturally low in saturated fats.

Application:
1. **Weeknight Dinner:** Serve Vegetarian Chili with Black Beans as a quick and nutritious weeknight dinner.
2. **Game Day or Potluck:** Prepare a batch for game day gatherings or potluck dinners.
3. **Meal Prep:** Make a larger batch and portion it for easy and healthy meal prepping.
4. **Toppings Bar:** Set up a chili toppings bar with options like shredded cheese, sour cream, and tortilla strips for a fun dinner party idea.

Cucumber and Tuna Salad

Ingredients:

- 2 large cucumbers, thinly sliced
- 2 cans (5 oz each) tuna, drained
- 1/2 red onion, thinly sliced
- 1 cup cherry tomatoes, halved
- 1/4 cup Kalamata olives, pitted and sliced
- 1/4 cup feta cheese, crumbled (optional)
- 2 tablespoons extra-virgin olive oil
- 1 tablespoon red wine vinegar
- 1 teaspoon Dijon mustard
- Salt and pepper to taste
- Fresh dill or parsley for garnish

Instructions:

1. **Prepare Vegetables:**
   - In a large bowl, combine thinly sliced cucumbers, red onion, cherry tomatoes, and Kalamata olives.
2. **Add Tuna:**
   - Gently fold in the drained tuna, breaking it into chunks.
3. **Make Dressing:**
   - In a small bowl, whisk together olive oil, red wine vinegar, Dijon mustard, salt, and pepper.
4. **Combine and Toss:**
   - Pour the dressing over the cucumber and tuna mixture.
   - Toss everything gently to coat the ingredients evenly.

5. **Optional Feta Topping:**
   - If desired, sprinkle crumbled feta cheese over the salad for an extra burst of flavor.
6. **Chill and Marinate:**
   - Cover the bowl and refrigerate for at least 15-20 minutes to allow the flavors to meld.
7. **Serve:**
   - Before serving, garnish with fresh dill or parsley.

Benefits:
   - **Rich in Omega-3s:** Tuna provides heart-healthy omega-3 fatty acids.
   - **Hydration:** Cucumbers contribute to hydration with their high water content.
   - **Protein Source:** Tuna offers a lean and satisfying source of protein.
   - **Vitamins and Minerals:** Vegetables like tomatoes and olives provide essential vitamins and minerals.

Application:
1. **Lunch Option:** Enjoy Cucumber and Tuna Salad as a light and nutritious lunch.
2. **Picnic or Potluck:** Pack this salad for a refreshing addition to picnics or potluck gatherings.
3. **Healthy Snack:** Serve as a healthy and satisfying afternoon snack.

4. **Summer Entertaining:** Include it in your summer menu for a cool and refreshing dish.

Caprese Skewers

Ingredients:
- 1 pint cherry tomatoes
- 1 package (about 8 ounces) fresh mozzarella balls (bocconcini)
- Fresh basil leaves
- Balsamic glaze for drizzling
- Extra-virgin olive oil for drizzling
- Salt and pepper to taste
- Wooden skewers

Instructions:
1. **Prepare Ingredients:**
   - Wash cherry tomatoes and pat them dry.
   - Drain the mozzarella balls.
2. **Assemble Skewers:**
   - Thread a cherry tomato onto a skewer, followed by a mozzarella ball, and a fresh basil leaf.
   - Repeat the pattern until each skewer is filled, leaving a bit of space at the ends for easy handling.
3. **Drizzle with Olive Oil:**
   - Arrange the skewers on a serving platter.
   - Drizzle extra-virgin olive oil over the skewers.

4. **Season:**
   - Sprinkle salt and pepper to taste over the assembled Caprese skewers.
5. **Drizzle with Balsamic Glaze:**
   - Just before serving, generously drizzle balsamic glaze over the skewers for a sweet and tangy finish.
6. **Serve:**
   - Serve immediately and enjoy the vibrant flavors.

Benefits:
- **Antioxidants:** Tomatoes and basil provide antioxidants that support overall health.
- **Protein and Calcium:** Mozzarella is a good source of protein and calcium.
- **Heart-Healthy Fats:** Olive oil contributes monounsaturated fats, promoting heart health.
- **Low-Calorie Snack:** Caprese skewers are a satisfying and low-calorie snack option.

Application:
1. **Appetizer:** Serve Caprese Skewers as a delightful and elegant appetizer at parties or gatherings.
2. **Snack Tray:** Include them on a snack or charcuterie tray for a burst of freshness.

3. **Outdoor Events:** Ideal for picnics, barbecues, and outdoor events due to their easy-to-eat nature.
4. **Lunch Box:** Pack them in lunch boxes for a healthy and satisfying snack.

Sweet Potato and Chickpea Buddha Bowl

Ingredients:
For the Bowl:
- 2 medium sweet potatoes, peeled and diced
- 1 can (15 oz) chickpeas, drained and rinsed
- 1 tablespoon olive oil
- 1 teaspoon smoked paprika
- 1 teaspoon ground cumin
- Salt and pepper to taste
- 4 cups cooked quinoa or brown rice

For the Toppings:
- 2 cups mixed greens (kale, spinach, arugula)
- 1 avocado, sliced
- 1 cucumber, sliced
- 1/2 cup cherry tomatoes, halved
- 1/4 cup red onion, thinly sliced
- 1/4 cup hummus
- Sesame seeds and fresh cilantro for garnish

For the Dressing:
- 3 tablespoons tahini
- 2 tablespoons lemon juice
- 1 tablespoon maple syrup or honey
- 1 clove garlic, minced
- Salt and pepper to taste
- Water to thin, if needed

Instructions:

1. **Roast Sweet Potatoes and Chickpeas:**
   - Preheat the oven to 400°F (200°C).
   - Toss diced sweet potatoes and chickpeas with olive oil, smoked paprika, cumin, salt, and pepper.
   - Spread them on a baking sheet in a single layer and roast for 25-30 minutes or until sweet potatoes are tender and chickpeas are crispy, stirring halfway through.
2. **Prepare Dressing:**
   - In a small bowl, whisk together tahini, lemon juice, maple syrup or honey, minced garlic, salt, and pepper. If the dressing is too thick, thin it with water until desired consistency is reached.
3. **Assemble Buddha Bowl:**
   - Divide cooked quinoa or brown rice among serving bowls.
   - Top with roasted sweet potatoes and chickpeas.
4. **Add Toppings:**
   - Arrange mixed greens, avocado slices, cucumber, cherry tomatoes, and red onion on top.
5. **Drizzle with Dressing:**
   - Drizzle the tahini dressing over the bowl.

6. **Garnish:**
   - Garnish with hummus, sesame seeds, and fresh cilantro.

Benefits:
- **Rich in Fiber:** Sweet potatoes and chickpeas provide dietary fiber, supporting digestive health.
- **Plant-Based Protein:** Chickpeas are a good source of plant-based protein.
- **Vitamins and Minerals:** The variety of vegetables offer essential vitamins and minerals.
- **Healthy Fats:** Avocado and tahini contribute heart-healthy monounsaturated fats.

Application:
1. **Lunch or Dinner:** Enjoy this Buddha bowl as a filling and nutritious lunch or dinner option.
2. **Meal Prep:** Prepare components in advance for easy meal prepping throughout the week.
3. **Potluck or Gathering:** Serve at potlucks or gatherings for a colorful and healthful dish.
4. **Customizable:** Customize with your favorite vegetables, grains, or proteins for variety.

Turkey and Vegetable Lettuce Wraps

Ingredients:
For the Filling:
- 1 pound ground turkey
- 1 tablespoon olive oil
- 1 onion, finely chopped
- 2 bell peppers (any color), diced
- 1 zucchini, diced
- 2 cloves garlic, minced
- 1 tablespoon soy sauce
- 1 tablespoon hoisin sauce
- 1 teaspoon ginger, grated
- 1 teaspoon sesame oil
- Salt and pepper to taste

For the Lettuce Wraps:
- Large lettuce leaves (such as iceberg or butter lettuce)
- Optional toppings: shredded carrots, sliced green onions, chopped cilantro, crushed peanuts

Instructions:
1. **Prepare Vegetables:**
   - Heat olive oil in a large skillet over medium heat.
   - Add chopped onion, bell peppers, zucchini, and minced garlic. Sauté until vegetables are softened.

2. **Cook Turkey:**
   - Push the vegetables to the side of the skillet and add ground turkey. Cook until browned and cooked through.
3. **Season and Sauce:**
   - Combine turkey with sautéed vegetables.
   - Add soy sauce, hoisin sauce, grated ginger, sesame oil, salt, and pepper. Stir to combine and let it cook for an additional 2-3 minutes.
4. **Assemble Lettuce Wraps:**
   - Spoon the turkey and vegetable mixture into large lettuce leaves, creating wraps.
5. **Add Toppings:**
   - Top each wrap with shredded carrots, sliced green onions, chopped cilantro, and crushed peanuts if desired.
6. **Serve:**
   - Arrange the lettuce wraps on a serving platter and serve immediately.

Benefits:
- **Lean Protein:** Ground turkey is a lean source of protein.
- **Vegetable Rich:** Bell peppers, zucchini, and onions provide vitamins and minerals.

- **Low-Carb Option:** Lettuce leaves replace traditional wraps, making this dish lower in carbs.
- **Flavorful Sauce:** Soy sauce, hoisin sauce, and sesame oil add depth and flavor to the filling.

Application:

1. **Healthy Lunch or Dinner:** Enjoy Turkey and Vegetable Lettuce Wraps as a light and healthy lunch or dinner option.
2. **Appetizer:** Serve them as appetizers at parties or gatherings.
3. **Meal Prep:** Prepare the filling in advance for quick and easy meal prepping.
4. **Customizable:** Customize the toppings and sauces based on personal preferences.

Greek Yogurt Parfait

Ingredients:

- 2 cups Greek yogurt (unsweetened)
- 1 cup granola (homemade or store-bought)
- 1 cup mixed berries (strawberries, blueberries, raspberries)
- 2 tablespoons honey or maple syrup
- 1/4 cup nuts (such as almonds or walnuts), chopped
- 1 teaspoon vanilla extract (optional)
- Fresh mint leaves for garnish (optional)

Instructions:

1. **Prepare Yogurt:**
   - In a bowl, mix Greek yogurt with vanilla extract if using. Set aside.
2. **Assemble Parfait:**
   - In serving glasses or bowls, layer the Greek yogurt, granola, and mixed berries.
3. **Repeat Layers:**
   - Repeat the layers until the glasses are filled, ending with a layer of mixed berries on top.
4. **Drizzle with Honey or Maple Syrup:**
   - Drizzle honey or maple syrup over the top of the parfait for added sweetness.

5. **Garnish:**
   - Garnish with chopped nuts and fresh mint leaves for added texture and flavor.
6. **Serve:**
   - Serve immediately and enjoy your delicious Greek Yogurt Parfait!

Benefits:
- **Protein-Rich:** Greek yogurt is a high-protein dairy product, promoting satiety.
- **Fiber and Nutrients:** Granola provides fiber and essential nutrients.
- **Antioxidant-Rich:** Berries offer antioxidants that support overall health.
- **Heart-Healthy Fats:** Nuts contribute healthy fats beneficial for heart health.

Application:
1. **Breakfast Option:** Greek Yogurt Parfait makes for a nutritious and satisfying breakfast.
2. **Snack:** Enjoy it as a wholesome and energizing snack.
3. **Dessert Alternative:** Serve as a healthier dessert option after meals.
4. **Brunch or Buffet:** Include in brunch spreads or dessert buffets for a crowd-pleasing treat.

Cauliflower Rice Pilaf

Ingredients:

- 1 large head of cauliflower, grated or processed into rice-like texture
- 2 tablespoons olive oil
- 1 onion, finely chopped
- 2 cloves garlic, minced
- 1 carrot, finely diced
- 1/2 cup peas (fresh or frozen)
- 1/4 cup chopped almonds or pine nuts
- 1 teaspoon ground cumin
- 1 teaspoon ground coriander
- Salt and pepper to taste
- Fresh parsley or cilantro for garnish
- Lemon wedges for serving

Instructions:

1. **Prepare Cauliflower Rice:**
   - Grate the cauliflower head or process it in a food processor until it resembles rice. Set aside.

2. **Sauté Aromatics:**
   - In a large skillet, heat olive oil over medium heat.
   - Add chopped onion and sauté until translucent. Add minced garlic and cook for an additional 1-2 minutes until fragrant.

3. **Add Vegetables and Nuts:**
   - Stir in finely diced carrot, peas, and chopped almonds or pine nuts. Cook

for 3-4 minutes until the vegetables are tender.

4. **Incorporate Cauliflower Rice:**
   - Add the cauliflower rice to the skillet, mixing well with the other ingredients.
5. **Season:**
   - Sprinkle ground cumin, ground coriander, salt, and pepper over the cauliflower rice. Stir to combine.
6. **Cook Until Tender:**
   - Cook for an additional 5-7 minutes, stirring occasionally, until the cauliflower rice is tender but not mushy.
7. **Garnish and Serve:**
   - Garnish the cauliflower rice pilaf with fresh parsley or cilantro.
   - Serve hot with lemon wedges on the side.

Benefits:
- **Low-Carb Alternative:** Cauliflower rice is a low-carb substitute for traditional rice.
- **Rich in Nutrients:** Cauliflower provides vitamins C and K, and is a good source of fiber.
- **Heart-Healthy Fats:** Olive oil and nuts contribute monounsaturated fats.
- **Vegetable Goodness:** Carrots and peas add color and additional nutrients.

Application:
1. **Side Dish:** Serve Cauliflower Rice Pilaf as a flavorful side dish alongside grilled chicken, fish, or tofu.
2. **Main Course:** Bulk it up with added protein like chickpeas or diced chicken for a satisfying main course.
3. **Meal Prep:** Prepare a batch for meal prepping and enjoy throughout the week.
4. **Vegetarian Option:** Make it a complete vegetarian dish by adding extra vegetables or tofu.

Shrimp Stir-Fry with Broccoli and Bell Peppers

Ingredients:
- 1 pound large shrimp, peeled and deveined
- 2 cups broccoli florets
- 1 red bell pepper, thinly sliced
- 1 yellow bell pepper, thinly sliced
- 3 tablespoons soy sauce
- 2 tablespoons oyster sauce
- 1 tablespoon hoisin sauce
- 1 tablespoon sesame oil
- 2 tablespoons vegetable oil
- 3 cloves garlic, minced
- 1 tablespoon ginger, grated
- 1 teaspoon cornstarch (optional, for thickening)
- Cooked rice or noodles for serving
- Sesame seeds and sliced green onions for garnish

Instructions:
1. **Prepare Shrimp:**
   - Pat the shrimp dry and season with salt and pepper.
2. **Stir-Fry Shrimp:**
   - Heat vegetable oil in a wok or large skillet over high heat.
   - Add shrimp and stir-fry for 2-3 minutes until they turn pink and

opaque. Remove shrimp from the wok and set aside.

3. **Sauté Vegetables:**
   - In the same wok, add a bit more oil if needed.
   - Add minced garlic and grated ginger, sauté for 30 seconds until fragrant.
   - Add sliced bell peppers and broccoli florets. Stir-fry for 3-4 minutes until vegetables are tender-crisp.

4. **Combine Shrimp and Vegetables:**
   - Return the cooked shrimp to the wok with the vegetables.

5. **Prepare Sauce:**
   - In a small bowl, whisk together soy sauce, oyster sauce, hoisin sauce, and sesame oil.

6. **Add Sauce to Stir-Fry:**
   - Pour the sauce over the shrimp and vegetables. Toss everything together to coat evenly.

7. **Optional Thickening:**
   - If you prefer a thicker sauce, mix 1 teaspoon of cornstarch with 1 tablespoon of water. Stir it into the sauce, and cook for an additional minute until it thickens.

8. **Serve:**
   - Serve the shrimp stir-fry over cooked rice or noodles.

- Garnish with sesame seeds and sliced green onions.

Benefits:
- **Lean Protein:** Shrimp provides a low-fat source of protein.
- **Vitamins and Fiber:** Broccoli and bell peppers offer essential vitamins and fiber.
- **Flavorful Sauce:** The combination of soy sauce, oyster sauce, and hoisin sauce adds depth and richness to the stir-fry.
- **Heart-Healthy Fats:** Sesame oil contributes heart-healthy monounsaturated fats.

Application:
1. **Quick Dinner Option:** Shrimp Stir-Fry with Broccoli and Bell Peppers is perfect for a quick and delicious weeknight dinner.
2. **Meal Prep:** Prepare ahead for easy meal prepping and enjoy throughout the week.
3. **Low-Carb Option:** Serve over cauliflower rice for a low-carb alternative.
4. **Family-Friendly:** A crowd-pleaser for family dinners or gatherings.

Egg and Spinach Breakfast Muffins

Ingredients:

- 6 large eggs
- 1 cup fresh spinach, chopped
- 1/2 cup red bell pepper, finely diced
- 1/2 cup onion, finely chopped
- 1/2 cup cherry tomatoes, diced
- 1/2 cup feta cheese, crumbled
- 1 teaspoon olive oil
- Salt and pepper to taste
- Cooking spray or muffin liners

Instructions:

1. **Preheat Oven:**
   - Preheat the oven to 375°F (190°C). Grease a muffin tin with cooking spray or use muffin liners.
2. **Sauté Vegetables:**
   - In a skillet, heat olive oil over medium heat.
   - Add chopped onion and diced red bell pepper. Sauté until softened.
3. **Add Spinach and Tomatoes:**
   - Add chopped spinach and diced cherry tomatoes to the skillet. Cook for an additional 2-3 minutes until the spinach wilts.

4. **Prepare Muffin Tin:**
   - Distribute the sautéed vegetable mixture evenly among the muffin cups.
5. **Crack Eggs:**
   - Crack one egg into each muffin cup over the vegetables.
6. **Season and Top:**
   - Season each egg with salt and pepper to taste.
   - Sprinkle crumbled feta cheese over the top of each muffin cup.
7. **Bake:**
   - Bake in the preheated oven for 15-20 minutes or until the egg whites are set, and the yolks are cooked to your liking.
8. **Cool and Serve:**
   - Allow the muffins to cool slightly before removing them from the tin.
   - Serve warm and enjoy your Egg and Spinach Breakfast Muffins!

Benefits:
- **Protein-Rich:** Eggs provide a high-quality source of protein.
- **Vegetable Nutrients:** Spinach, bell pepper, and tomatoes offer essential vitamins and minerals.
- **Healthy Fats and Calcium:** Feta cheese contributes healthy fats and calcium.

- **Low-Carb and Gluten-Free:** This recipe is suitable for low-carb and gluten-free diets.

Application:
1. **Quick Breakfast:** Egg and Spinach Breakfast Muffins are perfect for a quick and nutritious breakfast on busy mornings.
2. **Brunch Option:** Serve these muffins at brunch gatherings or potluck events.
3. **Meal Prep:** Make a batch during meal prep for convenient grab-and-go breakfasts throughout the week.
4. **Healthy Snack:** Enjoy them as a satisfying and healthy snack.

Salmon and Asparagus Foil Packets

Ingredients:
- 4 salmon fillets (6 oz each)
- 1 bunch asparagus, trimmed
- 1 lemon, thinly sliced
- 4 cloves garlic, minced
- 4 tablespoons olive oil
- 2 teaspoons Dijon mustard
- 1 teaspoon honey
- 1 teaspoon dried dill (or 1 tablespoon fresh dill)
- Salt and pepper to taste
- Fresh parsley for garnish
- Optional: Red pepper flakes for a hint of spice

Instructions:
1. **Preheat Oven:**
   - Preheat the oven to 400°F (200°C).
2. **Prepare Foil Packets:**
   - Cut four large pieces of aluminum foil. Place a salmon fillet in the center of each piece.
3. **Arrange Vegetables:**
   - Divide the trimmed asparagus evenly among the foil packets, arranging them alongside the salmon.

4. **Make Sauce:**
   - In a small bowl, whisk together minced garlic, olive oil, Dijon mustard, honey, dried dill, salt, and pepper.
5. **Drizzle Sauce:**
   - Drizzle the sauce over each salmon fillet and asparagus, ensuring they are well coated.
6. **Add Lemon Slices:**
   - Place a couple of lemon slices on top of each salmon fillet.
7. **Seal Packets:**
   - Fold the foil over the salmon and asparagus, sealing the edges to create packets.
8. **Bake:**
   - Place the foil packets on a baking sheet and bake in the preheated oven for 15-20 minutes or until the salmon is cooked through and flakes easily with a fork.
9. **Garnish and Serve:**
   - Carefully open the foil packets, garnish with fresh parsley, and serve the Salmon and Asparagus Foil Packets directly in the foil for easy cleanup.

Benefits:
- **Omega-3 Fatty Acids:** Salmon is rich in omega-3 fatty acids, supporting heart and brain health.
- **Vitamins and Minerals:** Asparagus provides essential vitamins and minerals, including folate and vitamin K.
- **Antioxidants:** Garlic, lemon, and dill contribute antioxidants that promote overall well-being.
- **Healthy Fats:** Olive oil offers monounsaturated fats, beneficial for heart health.

Application:
1. **Weeknight Dinner:** Salmon and Asparagus Foil Packets make for a quick and flavorful weeknight dinner.
2. **Outdoor Grilling:** Cook these foil packets on the grill for a delicious outdoor dining experience.
3. **Meal Prep:** Prepare several foil packets in advance for easy and convenient meal prepping.
4. **Special Occasions:** Serve this dish for special occasions or dinner parties for an impressive yet simple meal.

Mediterranean Quinoa Bowl

Ingredients:

For the Quinoa:
- 1 cup quinoa, rinsed
- 2 cups water or vegetable broth
- 1/2 teaspoon salt

For the Bowl:
- 1 can (15 oz) chickpeas, drained and rinsed
- 1 cup cherry tomatoes, halved
- 1 cucumber, diced
- 1/2 red onion, finely chopped
- 1/2 cup Kalamata olives, pitted and sliced
- 1/2 cup crumbled feta cheese
- Fresh parsley, chopped, for garnish

For the Dressing:
- 1/4 cup extra-virgin olive oil
- 2 tablespoons red wine vinegar
- 1 teaspoon dried oregano
- Salt and pepper to taste
- Optional: Garlic, minced, for added flavor

Instructions:

1. **Cook Quinoa:**
   - In a medium saucepan, combine quinoa, water or vegetable broth, and salt.
   - Bring to a boil, then reduce heat, cover, and simmer for 15-20 minutes, or until the quinoa is cooked and water is absorbed.

- Fluff with a fork and set aside to cool.
2. **Prepare Chickpeas:**
   - In a skillet, heat a bit of olive oil over medium heat.
   - Add chickpeas and cook for 5-7 minutes until they are slightly crispy. Set aside.
3. **Assemble Bowl:**
   - In serving bowls, arrange cooked quinoa, chickpeas, cherry tomatoes, diced cucumber, chopped red onion, Kalamata olives, and crumbled feta cheese.
4. **Make Dressing:**
   - In a small bowl, whisk together olive oil, red wine vinegar, dried oregano, salt, and pepper. Add minced garlic if desired.
5. **Drizzle Dressing:**
   - Drizzle the dressing over the quinoa bowl ingredients.
6. **Garnish and Serve:**
   - Garnish with fresh chopped parsley.
   - Toss everything together just before serving.

Benefits:
- **Plant-Based Protein:** Quinoa and chickpeas provide a hearty dose of plant-based protein.

- **Healthy Fats:** Olive oil and feta cheese contribute heart-healthy monounsaturated fats.
- **Rich in Antioxidants:** Tomatoes, olives, and red onion offer antioxidants for overall health.
- **Nutrient-Dense:** The bowl is packed with essential vitamins, minerals, and fiber.

Application:

1. **Lunch or Dinner:** Enjoy the Mediterranean Quinoa Bowl as a light and satisfying lunch or dinner option.
2. **Meal Prep:** Prepare components in advance for convenient and healthy meal prepping.
3. **Potluck or Gathering:** Bring it to potlucks or gatherings as a nutritious and flavorful dish.
4. **Customizable:** Add grilled chicken, shrimp, or additional vegetables to customize the bowl to your liking.

Grilled Chicken Breast with Lemon and Herbs

Ingredients:
- 4 boneless, skinless chicken breasts
- Zest and juice of 1 lemon
- 3 tablespoons olive oil
- 2 cloves garlic, minced
- 1 teaspoon dried oregano
- 1 teaspoon dried thyme
- Salt and pepper to taste
- Fresh herbs (such as parsley or rosemary) for garnish

Instructions:
1. **Marinate Chicken:**
   - In a bowl, combine lemon zest, lemon juice, olive oil, minced garlic, dried oregano, dried thyme, salt, and pepper. Mix well to create the marinade.

2. **Prepare Chicken:**
   - Pat the chicken breasts dry with paper towels.
   - Place the chicken breasts in a shallow dish and pour the marinade over them, ensuring each piece is coated. Marinate for at least 30 minutes, or refrigerate for up to 24 hours for more flavor.

3. **Preheat Grill:**

- Preheat the grill to medium-high heat.

4. **Grill Chicken:**
   - Remove the chicken from the marinade and let any excess drip off.
   - Grill the chicken breasts for about 6-8 minutes per side, or until the internal temperature reaches 165°F (74°C) and the chicken is no longer pink in the center.

5. **Rest and Garnish:**
   - Allow the grilled chicken to rest for a few minutes before serving.
   - Garnish with fresh herbs, additional lemon slices, and a drizzle of olive oil if desired.

Benefits:
- **Lean Protein:** Chicken breast is a lean source of high-quality protein.
- **Vitamin C:** Lemon provides a boost of vitamin C, supporting the immune system.
- **Heart-Healthy Fats:** Olive oil contributes monounsaturated fats beneficial for heart health.
- **Antioxidants:** Herbs add antioxidants, promoting overall well-being.

Application:

1. **Main Course:** Serve Grilled Chicken Breast as the main course for a light and flavorful dinner.
2. **Salads:** Slice grilled chicken and add it to salads for a protein boost.
3. **Sandwiches or Wraps:** Use grilled chicken in sandwiches or wraps for a tasty and healthy lunch option.
4. **Meal Prep:** Prepare extra grilled chicken for meal prepping and use it throughout the week in various dishes.

Avocado and Tomato Salad

Ingredients:

- 3 ripe avocados, diced
- 2 cups cherry tomatoes, halved
- 1/2 red onion, thinly sliced
- 1/4 cup fresh cilantro or parsley, chopped
- 1-2 tablespoons extra-virgin olive oil
- 1 tablespoon balsamic vinegar
- Juice of 1 lime or lemon
- Salt and pepper to taste
- Optional: Feta cheese or mozzarella, crumbled, for added creaminess

Instructions:

1. **Prepare Ingredients:**
   - Dice the avocados and halve the cherry tomatoes.
   - Thinly slice the red onion and chop the fresh cilantro or parsley.
2. **Assemble Salad:**
   - In a large salad bowl, combine the diced avocados, halved cherry tomatoes, sliced red onion, and chopped cilantro or parsley.
3. **Make Dressing:**
   - In a small bowl, whisk together extra-virgin olive oil, balsamic vinegar, lime or lemon juice, salt, and pepper.
4. **Drizzle Dressing:**

- Drizzle the dressing over the avocado and tomato mixture.

5. **Gently Toss:**
   - Gently toss the salad to ensure all ingredients are coated with the dressing.

6. **Optional Cheese:**
   - If desired, sprinkle crumbled feta cheese or mozzarella over the salad for added creaminess.

7. **Serve:**
   - Serve immediately and enjoy your refreshing Avocado and Tomato Salad!

Benefits:
- **Heart-Healthy Fats:** Avocados provide monounsaturated fats, which are beneficial for heart health.
- **Rich in Antioxidants:** Tomatoes and fresh herbs offer antioxidants that support overall well-being.
- **Vitamins and Minerals:** Avocados are a good source of vitamins E, C, B6, folate, and potassium.
- **Fiber:** This salad is rich in dietary fiber, promoting digestive health.

Application:
1. **Side Dish:** Serve Avocado and Tomato Salad as a vibrant side dish with grilled chicken, fish, or other main courses.

2. **Summer Picnics:** Pack this refreshing salad for summer picnics or beach outings.
3. **Taco Topping:** Use it as a topping for tacos or as a side for Mexican-inspired dishes.
4. **Lunch Option:** Enjoy the salad as a light and satisfying lunch on its own or with a piece of crusty bread.

CONCLUSION

By the time you finish the "Fast Feast Repeat Cookbook," we hope that the process of adopting a lifestyle that combines the benefits of a variety of delectable meals with the principles of Delay, Don't Deny Intermittent Fasting has inspired and delighted you.

This cookbook is more than simply a list of recipes; it's a manual for eating in a conscious, balanced manner where every mouthful is a celebration of good health.

We've worked hard to bring you a range of tasty and nourishing dishes in these pages that will satisfy both your fasting and feasting needs. This cookbook is based on the idea that feeding your body shouldn't be a chore but rather a delicious experience that improves your taste buds and your quality of life.

We urge you to cherish every meal, savor every moment, and recognize the benefits of mindful eating for your general wellbeing as you proceed on your path to a better and more conscious existence.

The recipes in these pages are designed to improve your fasting experience and turn every feast into a joyful occasion, whether you're looking for a simple and filling breakfast, a hearty lunch, or a delicious evening.

Recall that the "Fast. Feast. Repeat." rhythm is about more than just sticking to a plan; it's also about developing a healthy connection with food and creating a sense of balance that suits your particular requirements and tastes.

We hope that as you peruse the wide variety of recipes offered, you will uncover a world of gastronomic delights that perfectly complement your intermittent fasting lifestyle.

We are grateful that you let us share in your adventure. I hope you have plenty of food to go around, delicious feasts, and ongoing success in your efforts to become a healthier version of yourself. Toast to living life to the fullest, one delectable, well-balanced meal at a time!